Homemade Deodorant

How to Make Your Own Homemade Deodorant

(The Perfect Guide to Help You Make Your Own Natural Deodorant)

Maxine Hollis

Published By **Bella Frost**

Maxine Hollis

All Rights Reserved

Homemade Deodorant: How to Make Your Own Homemade Deodorant (The Perfect Guide to Help You Make Your Own Natural Deodorant)

ISBN 978-1-77485-659-8

Legal & Disclaimer

The information contained in this ebook is not designed to replace or take the place of any form of medicine or professional medical advice. The information in this ebook has been provided for educational & entertainment purposes only.

The information contained in this book has been compiled from sources deemed reliable, and it is accurate to the best of the Author's knowledge; however, the Author cannot guarantee its accuracy and validity and cannot be held liable for any errors or omissions. Changes are periodically made to this book. You must consult your doctor or get professional medical advice before using any of the suggested remedies, techniques, or information in this book.

Upon using the information contained in this book, you agree to hold harmless the Author from and against any damages, costs, and expenses, including any legal fees potentially resulting from the application of any of the information provided by this guide. This disclaimer applies to any damages or injury caused by the use and application, whether directly or

Table Of Contents

Introduction 1

Chapter 1: The Difference Between
Homemade And Commercial Products 5

Chapter 2: Detoxify Your Armpits 9

Chapter 3: Homemade Deodorant Simple
Recipe 13

Chapter 4: Homemade Deodorant Spray 17

Chapter 5: Homemade Deodorant Stick. 21

Chapter 6: Mild Homemade Antiperspirant
Cream 24

Chapter 7: Homemade Odorant Made
With Probiotics 27

Chapter 8: Homemade Odorant For Those
Who Don't Like Baking Soda 30

Chapter 9: Homemade Pocket Deodorizer
.... 34

Chapter 10: Why Are We Using
Deodorants 37

Chapter 11: Risks We Face When We Buy From Stores 41

Chapter 12: Homemade Deodorant Spray 45

Chapter 13: Homemade Antiperspirant . 50

Chapter 14: Homemade Deodorant Stick 54

Chapter 15: Homemade Deodorant Cream 60

Chapter 16: Homemade Whitening Deodorant 64

Chapter 17: Homemade Deodorant Made With Baking Sugar 69

Chapter 18: Homemade Deodorant Tips 73

Chapter 19: Deodorant: What Is It? 138

Chapter 20: Detox The Armpits Firstly . 145

Chapter 21: Deodorant For Sensitive Skin 150

Chapter 22: Homemade Fragrant Deodorants 160

Chapter 23: Soothing Deodorants 168

Chapter 24: Baking Soda - Free 174

Introduction

This book will show you how to make your very own homemade deodorant.

Are you thinking of making your very own deodorant? Or, do you think it's impossible to make your own? Let me tell you, it's possible. All you need is a basic kitchen tool.

There are many harmful chemicals in deodorants, and some of them contain ingredients we aren't even familiar with. Aluminum chlorohydrate (a kind of aluminum sodium) is one ingredient found in most deodorants. This ingredient is used to fight sweat and stop perspiration. However a high level can lead to cancer or Alzheimer's. Breast cancer is more common in females than males. This because your breast tissue is connected to your armpits. Parabens are also present in commercial deodorants and act as a stabilizer. Parabens work in the same way estrogen. If you have too many of them on your skin, it can cause damage to your health.

Here are some of those ingredients in the commercially sold deodorants or antiperspirants.

Aluminum – Many deodorants and antiperspirants include this in their ingredient list. A lot of studies have shown that aluminum has been linked with serious health problems.

Paraben-This is a synthetic preservative/drug that is used in many cosmetics products. Because it contains estrogen, it can affect hormonal balance.

Phthalates- A second ingredient that could cause serious problems for your health. This ingredient is often found in cosmetics.

Triclsoan (a pesticide) - According to FDA's classification, this product is considered a pesticide.

Propylene Glycol- This can be very dangerous if taken in large quantities.

You can experiment with your own recipe, just as you would with homemade products. Your homemade deodorants will keep their form and texture best when stored in cool areas. You can also include essential oils in your recipe to get additional benefits.

Be careful when mixing the ingredients. Make sure that you do not have any allergies to the materials. It is a good idea to first do a skin test before you proceed.

There are many testimonials that show homemade deodorants are superior to commercial products. Some of these homemade deodorants are so natural and organic they can be eaten.

There are many recipes you can find online. I have however saved you the time of searching through all those. Instead, I have collected it all here. Because antiperspirants contain aluminum, these recipes are not intended to be used. You need to be careful with how your homemade deodorant stains your clothes. I hope you have great fun making your very own deodorant. Say goodbye to those stale armpits and hello to a fresher, cleaner you.

Chapter 1: The Difference Between Homemade and Commercial Products

If you're considering making your own natural deodorant, then you may have struggled with the decision to make it worth your time or buy the most expensive on the market and hope for an amazing result.

Homemade products are more labor-intensive and require more attention. For some, the cost of making a product is not worth the time. Some people, however, would rather spend significant time making their product themselves because they believe the value of the money saved is greater than the effort they put into it.

It will be a contentious issue when it comes down to the financial aspects, but there are still many reasons why people would prefer to make products from scratch.

If you're a big fan commercially available deodorants then why not try making your own. These expensive deodorants claim they offer long-lasting protection and they are antiperspirant. However, did you know that many of the chemicals that are used on deodorants could be harmful to your skin? The majority of deodorants on the market today contain harsh chemicals that can damage your skin and cause allergic reactions.

Shopping for skin care products should be done with a sense of humour. It is important to pay attention what you put on your skin, especially where it touches sensitive areas such as your armpits. If you see a product promising you antiperspirant, whitening, or long-lasting protection it is likely that it has undergone a lengthy process that involved a lot many chemicals.

Look out for products without chemicals. Or, if one isn't available, make your very own. Simply buy the ingredients and make your personal deodorant. The packaging may seem extravagant, but do you know what the process was to create these containers and labels?

There are many benefits to making your own homemade deodorant

Creative Mind - When you are free to use your imagination and try out different recipes until you find the right one, you're more creative. Making your own deodorant is the first step. Once you do that, you will make many more.

Eco-friendly – When you make your products yourself, you don't need to destroy any natural resources.

Self-reliance: You can practice independence and improve your resourcefulness.

Education – It is a great idea to continue learning and taking the time to study and research new topics.

Know the Ingredients - By learning the differences and benefits of each ingredient, you will be able to make more homemade products.

Chapter 2: Detoxify Your Armpits

This is the very first step to make homemade deodorants work for you. Many people have believed for many years that a commercially available, effective deodorant would eliminate body odor. This is incorrect. What happens if deodorant is forgotten to be applied? Are you going to get a bad odor from your body? My opinion is that you won't.

Your skin is one of the most important parts of your body. Anything put on it can easily enter your body. To eliminate the toxins on our skin and to pull out the chemicals, detoxification is a must at least once every year.

Is it possible to make it work?

It works. This is what I found out. These are the results

* No body odor at all, even if we don't use any deodorant.

* No one ever got irritation or rashes while using homemade deodorant.

* We noticed less sweat in the area around the armspits.

* We'd love to do detox again and highly recommend it.

What should I do?

It is the process of detoxifying that involves changing from a regular to an organic or natural deodorant. The goal is to remove dead skin tissue from years of continuous use and to eliminate chemical build-up.

Ingredients:

* Bentonite Clay (1 Tbsp.)

* Apple Cider Vinegar, or Lemon Juice (1 tsp.

* Water (1-2 Tablespoons).

Procedure:

Use a wooden spoon, ladle, or wooden ladle to combine all ingredients until you achieve a creamy consistency. If you are not comfortable with the vinegar aroma, lemon juice may be substituted.

Apply the lotion to your armpits with your hands. Allow it to sit for around 8-20 minutes. If the skin is irritated, wash it immediately.

You may notice some reddening on your skin. It is normal.

Use warm water or a cloth to clean the cloth.

* Repeat this every day for approximately one week, or until armpit odor stops and irritation from homemade perfume is gone.

It is important to detoxify our whole body, not just the armpits. We have been taught to believe that sweat must be avoided, and that the armpit should never smell stale. The odor from our armpits can be traced back to the products that we used. These chemicals have been built up over years and are now being eliminated by detox. Our sweat serves as a means for toxins from entering our bodies. It's safe enough to assume that sweat, if only natural and organic substances are applied to our armpits, we won't get any unwanted body smells. Because it doesn't contain any toxic chemicals, Remember that fewer harmful toxins is equivalent to fewer unpleasant odors.

Chapter 3: Homemade Deodorant Simple Recipe

Did you last check your medicine cupboard? How many deodorants do your cabinets have? There are many brands out there, but it can be hard for people to decide which one they should use. There are lots of recipes on the internet, but I will show you a very simple recipe that I know would make your job so much easier.

What you should know:

* Baking Soda (1/4 Cup).

* Cornstarch (or Arrowroot Powder) (1/4 Cup).

* Coconut Oil (6-8 Tablespoons)

What you should do

* Combine the baking powder and arrowroot or cornstarch.

* Add the coconut oils gradually to the bowl and mix well until it forms a thick consistency.

* Add more cornstarch if the mixture is still too runny.

* You can use them in used deodorant containers. This mixture can last up to three years.

* Essential oils may also be added to your pits to provide aromatherapy and additional moisture.

Are you going to smell?

Are you wondering if there will be body odor? I can guarantee that this simple and effective recipe will work miracles for your pits.

The recipe will not be antiperspirant.

There will be different effects for everyone. But this is normal because the body is used to branded perfumes and it reacts differently when using natural deodorants.

What to Expect

Itchiness/Rashes

The baking soda may cause some itching, or worse, you might get rashes. These rashes may disappear in a few short weeks. If they continue to persist, you may reduce baking soda by 1 teaspoon. By replacing it with more cornstarch and arrowroot powder.

Itchyness can also occur if the deodorant is applied right after shaving. You should wait for at least an hour before applying it. The recipe may include shea butter for healing benefits.

Olive Oil can you be used in place of it?

I'd suggest not as they tend to be liquidy in nature, making it messy. Coconut oil can be used because it stays solid. Palm oil can also work, although they do not retain as much heat as coconut oil.

Will my clothes get stained?

No, they're not. Some faint stains may be normal.

Cornstarch or Arrowroot Powder

We strongly recommend that arrowroot powder be used.

Chapter 4: Homemade Deodorant Spray

Some people prefer a spray, cream, or stick deodorant to other options. Spray deodorant dried faster than creams, roll-ons, or creams. Also, they don't leave any marks on your clothes. This is all down to personal preference.

I have a solution for anyone who is considering making their own deodorant. You will find a couple of easy recipes here to suit your preferences.

A simple home-made deodorant spray that is refreshing and easy to use

What you should know:

* Ethyl Alcohol (Do not use itopropyl [rubbing] because it can be toxic if it is used for a longer amount of time).

* Refillable Spray Bottle available at any personal homecare shop

* Essential Oils (Not Synthetic)

What to do

* Simply pour alcohol into the spray can.

* Add a couple essential oils to the alcohol to enhance aroma and provide additional benefits.

This recipe is simple and won't take much time. However, it will still provide you the same benefits a regular deodorant. While the deodorant will kill bacteria that causes bad body odors, the alcohol is not antiperspirant. You can find another recipe that has a lot more power, but not alcohol.

Natural Deodorant Spray - No Baking Soda/No Alcohol

What you should know:

* Magnesium oils (4 ounces).

* Essential Oils

Spray Bottle

What to do

* Add the magnesium oils to the spray bottles.

* Add essential oils to aromatize and get additional benefits

Spray a small amount underarm with the spray and let dry for around 5-10 seconds

A few people may feel a tingling sensation, especially if they are low in magnesium. But it will go away after one week of using the homemade deodorant. An apple cider vinegar rinse can be applied to the underarm after you shower to extend the effectiveness.

These two recipes will not stain clothes or leave oily marks. They don't require baking soda. However, they are very effective in eliminating germs and bacteria from your underarm. Magnesium olive oil is a good substitute for baking soda. It does exactly the same thing to your underarms as baking soda, but it doesn't trigger them. Additionally, even though it may feel oily, it doesn't contain any oil, which can cause your body to have more magnesium. These recipes can be used for people who prefer oil-free baking soda.

Make sure you only use organic and natural essential oils. These oils are more effective than synthetic oils and can cause allergic reaction. You may want to try lemongrass and litsea curbeba if your sweat is heavy. If you prefer a stronger smell, you might consider peppermint essential oils or lavender essential oils.

Chapter 5: Homemade Deodorant Stick

This homemade all natural deodorant will work well for the traditionalist who doesn't trust a traditional stick. Human skin is the largest body organ. Anything you put on it will easily find its ways into your body. Use of harsh chemicals on your skin can put you at higher risk of developing cancer.

This recipe can be used by people who don't want to pay as much for deodorant they make online. Another advantage to this recipe is that it doesn't melt. It also stays solid in the container, making it easier for you to apply it.

Al Natural Homemade Deodorant Stick

What you should know:

* Baking Powder (1/8 cup).

* Arrowroot Powder (1/2 Cup)

* Beeswax (1 heaping TBSP.

* Tea Tree Essential Oils (8 drops).

* Lavender Essential Oil (8 Drops)

* Castor Oil (2 drops).

* Other essential oils to create a pleasant fragrance

What to do

* Mix all ingredients under a very low flame.

* Melt all the ingredients. The beeswax may need to take a little longer to melt.

* Mix occasionally, making certain that all ingredients are thoroughly incorporated

* A slightly thick and creamy mixture will let you know it's done.

* Place it into a clean, empty container of deodorant. (Clean it with care).

* Mix the ingredients together in a container.

* Allow it stand for at least 2 hours to let it set. You can also put it in the fridge for faster results.

This recipe is for one container of average size. You may need to make more containers. While it won't hold up as well as regular deodorant in warmer climates, it will still last. Use it by twisting it high enough. It is best to only use a small amount on your underarm for the first few week. While it's tempting to do more, you should remember that this is a transitional period. For the first few weeks, only use a light amount until your underarms become accustomed to the new scent.

Chapter 6: Mild Homemade Antiperspirant Cream

This mild homemade cream deodorant will definitely hit the spot. Because it's not just deodorant, it also contains a cream to soothe irritation. This cream doubles for your underarm. After all that years of wearing regular deodorants containing a lot of harmful chemicals, you should have a messed up armpit.

Mild homemade deodorant

It's basically going to infuse two kinds of oils with herbs. This project will use sunflower and coconut oil, but you could also use other oils. The herbs will be calendula and camomile.

What you should know:

* Coconut Oil (0.5 Tbsp.

* Sunflower Oil (or other oil) (3 Tbsp.

* Baking soda (4 cups + 2 Tbsp.

* Arrowroot powder (1/4 cup + 2 Tbsp.)

* Dried Calendula (3 Tbsp)

* Dried Chamomile (3 Tablespoons)

* Essential Oils (maximum 10 drops)

What you do

* Dry calendula leaves or chamomile, then put them in an airtight container.

Then add the sunflower oil and coconut oil. Before you add the coconut oil to the jar make sure it is in liquid form.

* Cover the jar, and keep it in cool and dark for around 2-3 weeks. You should give it a shake once in a while.

* Infused herbs will now be beautiful yellow after about two weeks.

* Do not heat the infused mixture once it has set.

* Strain your oil by using a strainer.

* Keep the strainer in place on top of a bowl until all the oil has been drained.

* Keep at least 5 to 7 tablespoons of infused oils after.

* Stir the dry ingredients into the baking soda and arrowroot, then add them to the mixture.

* Put in your desired essential oils.

The mixture should be creamy and semi-thick. After that, the deodorant should last for approximately 3 to 6 months. Simply rub the cream onto your armpits. To avoid any contamination, please make sure the jar has been sterilized. I would strongly recommend using arrowroot Powder instead of cornstarch to minimize irritation.

Chapter 7: Homemade odorant made with probiotics

We will use probiotics. Probiotics aid in digestion and you may have heard about them in food products. Probiotics are found in food products and can be used to make homemade deodorant. This recipe is sure to please!

Probiotics are able to improve the balance of good bacteria and bad bacteria under your arms, similar to the way they balance your stomach. Studies have shown that it can offer great relief from skin diseases such as eczema. Skin allergies, psoriasis. rashes. It can also help to diminish those unsightly underarm wrinkles. Regular deodorants have antiperspirants. They kill bad bacteria that causes a foul-smelling body odor.

Probiotics in Homemade Deodorant

What you should know:

* Coconut Oil (1 tablespoon).

* Shea Butter (1 tsp.

* Cocoa Butter (1 Tbsp.)

* Baking Sda (1Tbsp.

* Beeswax (1 tablespoon)

* Essential oils (Maximum 15 drops).

* Vitamin-E Oil (1/4 tsp.)

* Powdered probiotics (2 capsules)

What you should do

* Melt the shea butter/cocoa butter and beeswax on low heat.

* Let the pan cool, then add the arrowroot powdered and baking soda slowly, making sure to incorporate it fully into the mixture.

* Add Vitamin E oil, and the essential oils.

* Let the pan cool for an hour or until it is fully cooled.

* Combine the ingredients in a deodorant container. Let it cool in the refrigerator.

The probiotic tablets that will be used for this recipe should be full of the right bacteria. If you have an allergy to baking soda, you can try arrowroot or just omit the baking soda.

Chapter 8: Homemade odorant for those who don't like baking soda

Some people who attempted to make homemade deodorants developed allergic reactions to baking powder. Other people experienced dry skin, dry skin, and skin rashes. I feel sorry for you if you are one of them. I have a couple recipes that don't require baking sugar, yet they are very effective.

Homemade Deodorant that doesn't contain Baking Sugar

What you should know:

* Virgin Coconut Oil (30g).

* Shea Butter (20g)

* Beeswax (20g).

* Tamanu Oil (22.5g).

* Neem Oil (22.5).

* Almond Oil (3g).

* Vitamin-E Oil (10-18 drops)

* Frankincense Essential Oil (30 Drops)

* Bergamot Essential Oil (10 drops)

* Patchouli Essential Oil (10 drops).

* Arrowroot Powder (22.5g)

* Diatomaceous (15g)

* Kaolin Clay (7.5g).

* Double Broiler

What to do

* Combine all the ingredients except for the essential oils, dry ingredients and vitamin-E in the top half of the double broiler. Stir continuously.

* Make sure that beeswax has fully melted

* Turn it off, and let the mixture rest for 30 to cool.

* Now, combine the dry ingredients with the vitamin-e/essential oils.

Mix thoroughly, and then transfer to the empty deodorant bottles.

This recipe is enough to fill two regular-sized deodorant cans. You might be wondering why this recipe has so many ingredients.

Neem Oil: This oil is very thick and has many uses. You can also use it as a repellant for bugs. This oil is antiseptic, bacterial, and antifungal.

Tamanu Oil- Some say it is a miraculous oil. This oil isn't well-known by many. Tamanu Oil may be a very effective oil for skin healing. This will be great for your underarm because it can help to regenerate those skin cells you've lost from regular deodorants over the years.

Shea Butter - This is a raw, unrefined form of shea butter that's very good for your skin.

Beeswax-This is a great stabilizer to any cosmetic recipe. It makes the mixture thicker. Beeswax can also help to retain moisture on your skin.

Arrowrot Powder - This is the main ingredient of any homemade deodorant. Because it thickens any recipe and draws out toxins.

Kaolin – A mild clay, which can help to get rid of any impurities under your arm.

Diatomaceous Erd - This ingredient draws out toxic substances and aids with sensitive skin.

Chapter 9: Homemade Pocket Deodorizer

Let's get to the bottom of this chapter and talk about my secret, which I always keep in my bag. This is my quick deodorizer. While you can apply make-up or perfumes, it does not make you feel confident. This small deodorizer makes you feel fresh again, ready to face any situation without having to think about your body odor.

It is evident that when you switch from a regular deodorant, to an all-natural, organic deodorant, you will notice some changes. You may also notice that your sweating is more intense. But this is just because your body is still adjusting. It might take a few months before your sweating normalizes. So while you wait, bring this portable deodorizer with to keep you fresh!

Pocket Deodorizer

What you should know:

* Vodka

* Distilled Water

* Essential Oil (Preferably antibacterial like lavender and tea trees)

What to do

* Use a small clean or spray bottle. Before using it, sterilize it.

* Combine equal parts of water with vodka.

* Add between 15-25 drops to your preferred essential oil.

* Combine all ingredients.

These are all the ingredients you need in order to make a body odor defense weapon. The vodka can dry out your underarm sweat and prevent any body or body odor. You should strongly consider using an antibacterial essential oil to help protect your body from unwanted odor.

Do not drink from the bottle. The essential oils will become inedible once they have been put into it. This bottle can dry your underarms and skin so do not use it very often.

Another great tip. If you do not have this bottle, you can order vodka with tonic, dip a piece of toilet paper or a washcloth, and sneak into the restroom. Once you're there, wipe the alcohol on your underarm. It will immediately stop the sweating.

Chapter 10: Why are we using deodorants

Personal hygiene is crucial for your body's health and well-being. Good hygiene is about having self-control and respecting yourself. A common problem with personal hygiene and grooming is body odor. B.O., as it is also known, is a sign of bacteria in the body. Research shows that bacteria in our skin can lead to body odor (B.O.). If you sweat frequently, bacteria in your skin can become active and multiply, leading to unpleasant odors.

The skin is made up different layers and has many glands. Some glands secrete liquids. They are also known as sweat cells. There are two types. Eccrine can be found everywhere in the body and control the body's temperature. Apocrine, on the other side, is mostly located in the armpits. These glands will be activated when the body feels anxious, nervous, stressed, or hot. Because the armpits can be moist and dark, bacteria has a natural breeding ground, creating body odor.

Manufacturers found a way of controlling and minimizing body odor by using antiperspirants and/or deodorants.

What is the Difference Between Antiperspirants And Deodorants

Deodorant helps to eliminate unpleasant odors. It helps to control and minimize the growth of bacteria on your skin. Deoderant can be used to mask unpleasant smells and produce a pleasant, fragrant fragrance. This means that they mask unpleasant odors. Deodorant does nothing to slow down sweating.

Antiperspirants, however, work by decreasing sweat levels. Antiperspirants can keep armpits clean and dry. They also help to control bacteria growth. Antiperspirants are considered deodorants, as they fulfill both functions.

Different bodies have different chemistries. Deodorant is not required by everyone. Deos are not necessary for everyone. Let me clarify: Some people sweat profusely. They need a product to help them stop looking terrible and avoid embarrassing others.

How can these products be applied or used?

There are many types of antiperspirant available on the market. They come in a variety of forms: creams, sprays (pump sprays), aerosol sprays; creams and sticks. To ensure the best results, follow the manufacturer's instructions. After a shower, apply the products to your arms and allow them to dry. So that the product does not stick to your clothing, allow it to dry. Avoid direct contact with your eyes when spraying.

No matter your reasons, deodorants can be useful for you. But it is important to learn how to use them properly and understand the health effects. But there's another way to get deodorants than buying them from the store. That is making your own. Continue reading and you will discover.

Chapter 11: Risks we face when we buy from stores

Deo is something that everyone needs to use, but there are some risks that we do not know about. You are also unknowingly risking your health by purchasing deodorant. Deodorants purchased in stores can pose some health risk due to the ingredients used and how they are made. Here are some examples.

Aluminum

It is easy to forget that the aluminum found in deodorants can cause serious health problems. Aluminum helps keep sweat from entering our pores, so almost all deodorants contain this ingredient. It is an ingredient in antiperspirant soaps. However, it can increase your risk of developing certain diseases, such as cancers of the breasts, kidney problems, seizures, and Alzheimer's.

Parabens

Parabens are a common preservative found in most personal care products. Parabens may disrupt our hormonal equilibrium, which can lead early puberty, higher chances of developing hormonal cancers, such as breast or cervical cancer, and even birth defects in pregnancies.

Propylene Glycol

This ingredient is also used in many other products, such as processed food. It speeds up the process of skin drying by absorbing quickly. It is a petroleum-based compound that is used in softening cosmetic products. Propylene glycol may damage our heart and liver, as well as our nervous systems, particularly the central.

Fragrances

Fragrances may conceal many chemicals like phthalates that can cause health problems. Fragrances have a higher risk of birth defects, as they disrupt hormone receptors which can lead to cell mutations.

Triclosan

This is most often used to kill bacteria. However the FDA classified it as pesticide. One that should not be used in products such deo. BHA, BHT

BHA or BHT are more commonly known. Butylated Hydroxytoluene causes hyperactivity among children. It is associated with neurotoxicity, cancer, allergies as well cellular level biochemical and hormonal changes.

Studies show that the majority of deodorants can raise your chances of getting breast cancer or Alzheimer's disease. Although we may be concerned about these potential health issues, do we really think we should stop using deodorants? No. There are always alternatives to everything. This is why we want to let everyone know that it's possible to make your own deodorant. You can even make your own deodorant. We are here for you to find that perfect deodorant. You can make it yourself, or you can buy it as a stick, spray, cream, antiperspirant, cream or cream. Use homemade deodorant for the same benefits without the health risks. You'll thank yourself for it later.

Chapter 12: Homemade Deodorant Spray

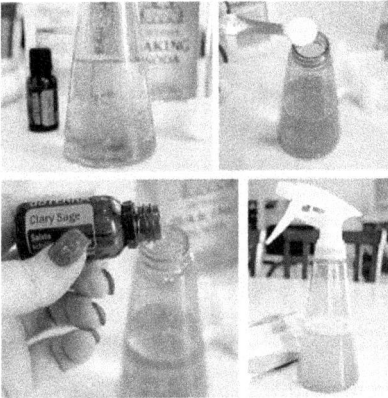

Are you tired using the same deodorant for both your perfume and your deodorant? Are you looking for a deodorant that also acts as a perfume? If so, why not create your own spray deodorant? Here's how:

Ingredients:

* 60ml distilled water

* 30ml vodka alcohol. Serves as a preservative. Also kills bacteria.

* 1 teaspoon rosewater

* 1 Tablespoon of magnesium oil

* 10 drops essential olive oil, preferably salvia Sclarea. Commonly known as Clary Sage oil.

* 4-8 drops each of grapefruit, lavender, and grapefruit essential oils. When mixed with tea oil, these essential oils create a strong fragrance.

* 4-8 drops (commonly referred to by tea tree oils) of melaleuca Oil, which kills germs underarms and causes body odor

* 1/2 cup of Hamamelis Virginiana, also known for Witch Hazel

* aloe vera Procedure:

1. First crush fresh rose petals and then use a mortar to make rose water. Prepare a sauce pan, then add enough water to cover the crushed petals. Boil the rose

water for about 10-15 minutes. Finally, allow it to cool, then filter the petals through a strainer.

2. For a tidy workspace, gather all necessary ingredients.

3. Next, you will need to make your own deodorant spray.

4. To prevent oil from dripping or overflowing, use a damp sponge to wipe the surface.

5. Put the distilled waters in a small mixing bowl. Next, add the vodka alcohol. Vodka prevents bacteria from causing odors. It also preserves homemade deodorant.

6. Add the rosewater, magnesium oil, and stir well. If you don't want to get a tingling sensation from magnesium oil, decrease its amount.

7. You can also add 10 drops Clary Sage essential ointment oil. This fragrance is

most effective at preventing strong body smells. Clary Sage essential oil can stimulate menstruation. Do not add Clary Sage essential oil to any pregnant woman. Clary Sage is sedative and should not be added to any alcohol-containing products. It is important to avoid applying this oil to low blood pressure as it may cause hypotension.

8. Finally, add 4-8 drops Teatree oil. This helps to reduce the underarm odor.

9. Make homemade deodorant by adding 4-8 drops of grapefruit oil extract, lemon oil, grapefruit oil extract, or geranium Oil Extract. These essential oils will work well with Tea tree and other oils.

10. Put in 1/2 cup of witch hzel. This helps keep your underarms dry and makes you feel fresh throughout the day.

11. Add the aloe extract, and stir the mixture well.

12. Make sure to shake the solution well before using it.

Making your own deo spray has two benefits. It can be used as a perfume or deo and also doubles up as a moisturizer. Only one spray is all it takes to smell fresh and stay hydrated.

Chapter 13: Homemade Antiperspirant

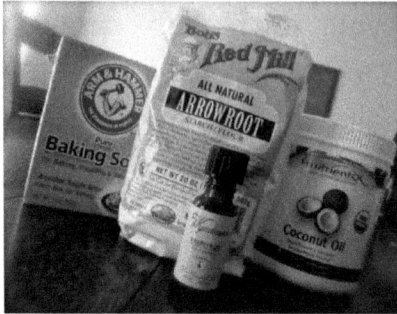

Many people hate when their armpits are covered in sweat. But many people avoid commercially prepared antiperspirants out of fear of contracting diseases or illnesses. Sometimes though, because there are no other options they either resort to using the antiperspirants that they have tried to avoid or suffer from sweaty underarms. You have the option to be different. Commercially made antiperspirants, deodorants, and deodorants can be said goodbye to aluminum and parabens.

These ingredients are believed to cause cancer. Because of this carefully designed homemade antiperspirant formula, these products are unlikely to come in contact with your skin.

Ingredients

* Organic shea or cocoa butter or organic mango butter (choose from any of these 3), 6 tablespoons

* Coconut oil, 2 tablespoons.

* Arrowroot powder, 1/4 cup

* Optional: Baking Soda Powder (choose the one without Aluminum), 4 teaspoons

* essential oils are rosemary, lavender or sage oil, or half a teaspoon.

Procedure

1. Use a glass bowl to combine all of your dry ingredients. These are the baking soda and arrowroot powder. Some people react

to baking soda with itchiness and red bumps. Mix them with a spatula (or a plastic lardle) until the mixture is consistent.

2. Heat your coconut oil and butter on low heat using a double oven. Don't boil. Mix the ingredients well. Then let cool.

3. When the mixture is cool enough, put it in a glass bowl. You can now mix the ingredients by holding a spoon or plastic ladle.

4. Add essential oils and oil, whichever option you have. To achieve the consistency you desire, make sure to mix in the oils slowly. The difference between a little bit of oil and a lot can be huge, so make sure to watch your portions.

5. Mix the ingredients together, and then seal it in a glass jar to extend its shelf life. Recycled glass jars can be used to store jams or peanut butter. You can also buy

ready-made glass jars and containers in DIY stores.

If you've tried many homemade natural antiperspirants from recipes online or received recommendations by friends, but you still haven't found one that works for you, this will be the perfect one. It is up to you how light or creamy your antiperspirant, as well the fragrances that it comes in. You can ensure it is not too heavy for your sensitive nose to absorb. It will instead make you love your homemade antiperspirant so much that you have to use it again and again until the essence disappears.

Chapter 14: Homemade Deodorant Stick

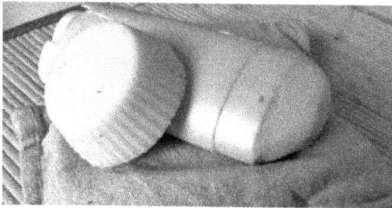

Use organic products to keep your skin fresh and beautiful. How to make your deodorant stick yourself Make your own homemade deodorant sticks and say good-bye to underarms that smell gross.

Ingredients:

* 1 Tablespoon Coconut Oil

* One and half tablespoons beeswax, to eliminate the underarm stink

* 1/3 cup of corn starch

* 1 fluid ounce (or more) of liquid chlorophyll. Helps to lessen unpleasant odors

* 0.7 ounces (20g), White Kaolin Clay - Keeps armpits sweat-free

* 12 cup cocoa butter

* 1/2 tablespoon shea Butter (refined or unrefined)

* 3-5 drops of castor oils - Lightens armpits that have darkened from shaving

* 10-15 drops White Thyme Essential Oil - Serves as an Antibacterial Component

* 10-15 drops of coriander oils - This helps prevent underarms and legs from perspiring

* 10-15 drops honeysuckle oil, lemongrass, teatree, or honeysuckle oil (anyone of the essential oils will suffice for fragrance).

* 20-25 drops essential oil of lavender
Procedure: You can gather all the necessary ingredients at a single counter to ensure a neat place and a continuous process.

2. For any spillages, drips or overflows that may occur, be sure to have a damp towel on hand.

3. To make the coconut oil, use a sauce pan or container made of ceramic, stainless, or ceramic. Add the 1 tablespoon of coconut oil and then the 1 1/2 tablespoons honey wax. Blend well, and let the wax mellow.

4. Once the beeswax melted, you can add 1/2 tablespoon cocoa butter or shea butter (either refined oder not). Gently mix the beeswax in with the cocoa and refined shea butter. Blend well. Keep the stove on a low heat to avoid overcooking. To prevent the ingredients sticking,

carefully mix the butters with the wax using a stainless bowl.

5. Once the ingredients are melted off the stove, switch it off and continue mixing them to form lumps. Then let the solution cool for a while before transferring.

6. Once the mixture was well-refined, prepare a clean, glass mixing bowl. Use a spatula and gently add the melted ingredients to the bowl.

7. Add 1/3 cup of white kaolin or corn starch to the mixing bowl. Mix with the melted ingredients until you get a creamy texture. (If you have a hard time working with the mixture, you can heat the mixture once more to achieve the desired paste texture.

8. Let's get on to the liquids. You will need 1 fluid ounces liquid chlorophyll. This liquid prevents pasty solutions from hardening.

9. Add 3-5 drops to the castor oil.

10. Mix in 10-15 drops of whitethyme in the glass bowl.

11. Use 10-15 drops lemongrass, honeysuckle, tea tree or rosemary oil. You can use any of the essential oils.

12. Add 20-25 drops de lavender oil. This essential oils has antimicrobial capabilities that will help you maintain clean underarms.

13. Blend the essential oils and the melted components thoroughly.

14. Use a deodorant stick container that is clean and empty to pour the mixture. Avoid spills and drips

15. Then close the deodorant stick box and place in a freezer to freeze for 20 min. Store it in a dry, cool area after 20 minutes.

Making your own deodorant is simple and safe. This organic stick won't make you smell bad.

Chapter 15: Homemade Deodorant Cream

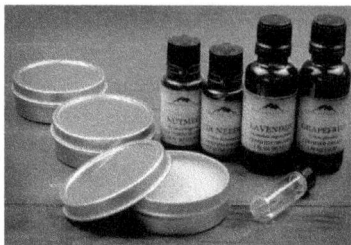

Homemade beauty and hygiene products are becoming more popular than commercially manufactured ones. Since some prefer deodorant creams creamy, all natural homemade products have been added to the variety of homemade beauty products. Here's a hand-picked recipe that doesn't include baking soda. This won't hurt especially when you apply it to your freshly shaved thighs.

Ingredients

* 1.4 ml of shea butter for its soothing skin effects

* 6 and 1/4 cups coconut oils - A strong, all-natural antibacterial agents

* To make the cream smooth and easy to apply, use 4 to 1/2 teaspoons beeswax.

* Sage essential oil – 3 drops is all it takes to make it antiperspirant

* Melaleuca essential ointment: Use 4 drops to add an additional antibacterial agent

* Lavender essential Oil - Use 8 drops to soothe and heal your skin after shaving.

* 5 drops vitamin E oil to extend shelf-life and increase antioxidant activity

Procedure

1. Prepare the ingredients, as well the utensils, that you will need to measure your ingredients. You should prepare your

container. You have two options: either you can buy a readymade 2 ounce container. It can be sterilized by heating water and then dried in the air.

2. Carefully measure the ingredients to ensure that they are proportioned according to the directions. It is important to not have too much or too small of any ingredient. This will result in a creamier product that meets the requirements for the application of deodorant crèmes. Don't forget that this is a deodorant cream. It is not a spray.

3. Combine all three ingredients, coconut oil, shea butter, and beeswax in a double burner and melt over low heat. Stir continuously until all three ingredients are completely melted. You'll end up with a smooth, even mixture. It is now time to remove from the heat and allow it to cool.

4. Add the essential oils (lavender and melaleuca) to the melted butter, coconut oil, beeswax and beeswax. It is important to accurately measure the ingredients to ensure that your homemade deodorant cream performs its function.

5. The prepared vitamin E should be added to the preparation in order to keep it fresh and stable for an extended shelf life. You should discard any preparation that appears out of place.

Your homemade deodorant cream recipe will ensure that you smell great every day. It has all of the necessary ingredients to make your homemade deodorant effective and prevent you from developing an unpleasant body odor. It can be used liberally and as often you require it. It's all-natural and contains no toxic chemical substances.

Chapter 16: Homemade Whitening Deodorant

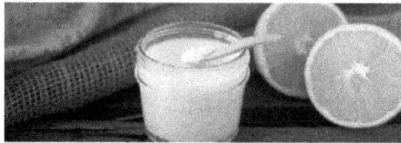

Dark underarms can be a burden on any woman. It limits her ability to wear what she likes. Do not let dark underarms stop you from trying different brands of deodorants. This chapter will show how to make your own.

Ingredients

* non GMO (Genetically Modified Organisms), cornstarch, arrowroot powderstarch

* Coconut oil

* vitamin E oil

* Lavender oil (or other essential oils used for scent)

* powdered orange skins

* Cocoa butter

* shea butter

Procedure

1. You should make powdered orange peels first. The strong citric acid content in orange skin contributes to its whitening capabilities. Use a peeler to remove the orange's skin. Once the orange rinds are peeled, place them on a piece if blanket and dry it for 4-6 hours.

Use a ceramic bowl to hold the peeled oranges. Place the bowl in an oven for at least 1 hour. You can take the bowl out from the oven with care and crush the dried orange skins using a mortar-and-pille.

2. Prepare the necessary kitchen utensils to measure out the ingredients used to make the homemade deodorant's base. It's easy to gather the ingredients.

3. A set of measuring spoons is all you need to scoop 1/2 tablespoon of cocoa or shea butter. Add the desired amount (this oil helps reduce unwanted underarm smells) to a ceramic saucepan. Then, add the small butter chunks. These butters will be broken up so turn down the heat on the kitchen stove to medium and use a stainless stirrer to thoroughly mix the shea/cocoa butter. Turn off the stove once the ingredients have melted. Blend the ingredients until you have a smooth mixture.

4. Prepare a large, glass mixing bowl. After the melted ingredients have been

incorporated, you will need to add the non GMO cornstarch/arrowroot starch. These ingredients keep sweat from your arms from getting into the starch. Use a stainless bowl to combine all ingredients until they are completely combined.

5. Once the mixture is refined, you can add 5 drops to your homemade whitening oil. You can also add 1 teaspoon vitamin E oil. This will make your underarm skin more healthy. Combine the oils and stir until they dissolve in the prepared mix.

6. You will want to keep a moist cloth handy in case you make a mess from the mixture spilling over or drippings.

7. Once you've mixed all the ingredients of your homemade whitening toothpaste, strain the mixture into the measuring cup.

8. You can pour the mixture from the measuring cups into clean and empty deodorant containers.

9. The mixture can be used for up to 4 2.6oz deodorant pots

You can make your own homemade whitening toothpaste. It's easy to make, and it is safer than buying commercial products.

Chapter 17: Homemade Deodorant made with Baking Sugar

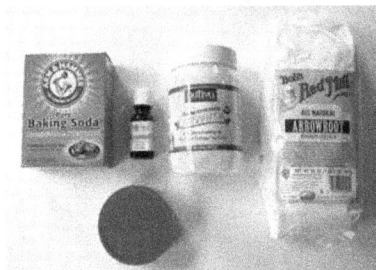

You have many options for natural ingredients to make homemade deodorant. Baking soda is an ingredient that's commonly found in most kitchens. It can be used to make batter mix and baking pastries. However, it can also be used to make your own deodorant recipe.

Baking soda, a replacement product for continuous sweating in the armpits, can help to prevent it. It absorbs moisture and is therefore useful because it has an antiperspirant feature.

Ingredients

14 cup baking soda

* 1/4 cup of arrowroot or cornstarch

* 5 tablespoons coconut butter

* Use your preferred essential oils

Procedure

1. Because we are discussing homemade recipes, it would make sense to make them eco-friendly. Consider buying a new container or canister. This is going to be easy for women since you have many cosmetic bottles that you don't need anymore. Get rid of all the product residue and wash the container. Use a towel to dry the container.

2. 1 cup of baking soda should be poured into the container. You do not need any particular brand of baking soap to make this recipe.

3. Stir in 1/4 cup of arrowroot paste after you have poured the baking soda. If arrowroot is unavailable, you can substitute cornstarch. Because it feels more natural on the skin than cornstarch and arrowroot, it is more beneficial. But, if you don't have arrowroot powder, you could always use cornstarch. Cornstarch comes in two options: talc free or untalc. These powders help reduce the sweat production. Also, the irritating effects caused by baking soda can be tempered with arrowroot and cornstarch powders.

4. Combine the baking soda and the cornstarch/arrowroot powder very well.

5. After you have mixed the ingredients, add in five tablespoons Coconut oil. Coconut oil can harden sometimes so heat it up on low heat until it melted completely. After cooling it, pour it into the mixture. It will burn the baking soda

and cornstarch if you abruptly pour it after heating it.

6. Lastly, add your desired essential oil. This is optional but you can add your essential oil. You can make an antiperspirant as well as a deodorant. Depending on your choice, you can use either two or four essential oils. Mixing essential oils is possible, but you should verify the label to confirm that it is legal. The essential oil concentration rate will determine the quantity of drops.

7. Mix all ingredients thoroughly. Once everything is well combined, seal the container and let it dry.

Making your own homemade recipe is simpler and more efficient than buying ready-made products. It only takes a few days to notice the difference.

Chapter 18: Homemade Deodorant Tips

Body odor is something that cannot be stopped. The secretion sweat is a natural part in the body's process. It is one method of removing unwanted substances from our system. However, we can control the smells of body odors. It is well-known that many antiperspirants and deodorants in the local markets contain harmful chemicals. These chemicals can cause skin irritations and allergies, particularly if your skin has sensitive areas.

Fearing that we might be irritated by commercial products, many homemade recipe lovers and enthusiasts continue to create new recipes. While there are many advantages to homemade recipe, we also have to acknowledge the downsides.

This chapter will examine the pros and cons of homemade deodorants.

Dos and Don'ts of Homemade Deodorant

You can use all-natural deodorants that include peppermint oil, tea tree oils, or lavender to reduce the growth of bacteria.

It is true that salt crystals should be avoided, but it all depends on how they are used. If you don't sweat a lot these crystals might be a good choice. Use salt crystals in combination with homemade deo or talc powder to make them effective.

Stick to simple, all-natural ingredients when creating your own recipes. Some of these ingredients can be found in your kitchen, while others are readily available at your local supermarkets. Many of these ingredients can be costly, especially essential oils. So make sure to use what you have on hand.

If you do not want to use alcohol in your homemade deodorant base, don't use it. It is scientifically proven to have skin-damaging effects. Use high-proof, ethyl ethanol instead.

Always refer to the label before you purchase organic ingredients. You need to be able to tell if the ingredient's concentration is high or low. It might hurt or sting if you have just shaved your arms.

Even if ingredients are organic they may not suit all skin types. You should first do a skin test and check for any adverse reactions.

The Don'ts of Using Homemade Deodorant

Make your homemade deodorants last for a while. It is important to continue using the homemade deodorants for at least three days. This will allow your skin to adjust. Your skin is familiar with the chemical components found in regular deodorants used for years. It takes time and effort to balance it.

Bake soda shouldn't be applied directly on the skin.

It is better to make your own recipes for your underarm problems.

What causes body odors?

This book will guide you through making homemade deodorants. You might be wondering why you would need to make your deodorant yourself when there are so many choices. Making your own deodorant means you have complete control over what you put in it.

Deodorant can be applied or sprayed on the body to eliminate foul-smelling odors that are caused by bacteria being broken down in different areas, like the feet and armpits. It is possible to use deodorant on many parts of the body. But, the antiperspirants group, which are usually found underarms, are used most frequently. Antiperspirants block sweat from the area they are applied. The Food and Drug Administration of the USA (FDA) places antiperspirants in the over-the–counter drug category. They also consider many of the available cosmetic deodorants to be cosmetics.

While using homemade deodorants is safer and easier than buying commercial ones, this does not disprove the widespread myth that the use of them can lead to breast cancer. This claim is not supported by any solid evidence.

The source of the foul stench?

Human sweat is actually non-obtrusive. It becomes odorless when it is exposed to bacteria. This occurs most commonly in environments that are hot and humid. The human body's underarms are the most consistently warm. The sweat glands produce water to cool your underarms.

As you age your skin, especially around your armpits becomes more susceptible for bacterial growth. This is caused by frequent washing the skin with an acid pH soap. This causes the acid mantle to slowly deteriorate and the skin pH to increase. Because bacteria feeds on sweat from the skin, they will often find dead hair and skin cells. During the process, the bacteria release waste that contains trans-3-Methyl-2-hexenoic acid. This is the main culprit for the foul odor.

Over-the-Counter Deodorants

The majority of deodorants on the market today are alcohol-based. Alcohol acts by temporarily stimulating sweat production and getting rid off bacteria. These deodorants can also include sodium chloride or stearyl Alcohol. There are also stronger options that combat bacterial growth such triclosan or other metal chelant substances. There are many deodorants with added ingredients like essential oils and perfumes. They will not get rid of the foul odor but mask it.

Antiperspirants

These products reduce sweating in your underarms and prevent bacteria from growing. These products usually contain aluminium chlorohydrate (aluminum chlorohydrate), aluminium-zirconium complexes and aluminium chloride. For the greatest benefits, you should apply these types of products before bed.

Concerns about Health

Zirconium deodorants can cause allergic reactions in some people. Others may experience irritations when using antiperspirants with proylene glycol. It is safer for sensitive skin to choose alcohol-free products

Preventing Body Odor

To maintain your health and protect yourself against various diseases, it is essential to have a healthy personal hygiene. Bromhidrosis, also known as body smell, is a condition that begins around puberty. This is because your system has more androgens. These hormones can only become active after you reach puberty. This is why body smell is not an issue for children. Your body regulates temperature by sweating. The sweat reacts to the bacteria on the skin's surface and produces a foul-smelling odor.

BO or body odor does not just occur in the arms. The bacteria can also thrive on other parts of the body, including the anus region (groin), upper thighs, feet and groin. Even though a bath can temporarily resolve the problem, it's not always the best solution. You can get smelly shoes, which can lead to stale feet. The shoes must be taken care of, in addition to hygiene. The same applies for your body. You must wear the right clothes.

These are the top tips to get rid of body odor.

1. Make sure your underarms are as dry as possible. It is important to remember that bacteria thrives in moist places, so don't give them any comfort by keeping your underarms dry.

2. Antiperspirant should be used if you tend to sweat a lot. This will allow the product work while you're asleep, so you don't have to sweat. The product should not be applied after a bath because your body will lose its ability to absorb the water and it will then need to be washed away.

3. Hyperhidrosis is a condition in which excessive sweating is common. This can be treated by visiting a doctor. You might not be aware that it could be caused by other

conditions. A professional can diagnose the problem and prescribe the appropriate medication.

4. This is the solution. It can be used at home to eliminate bacteria that causes the odor. It is composed of one cup water and three percent hydrogen peroxide. Only need to dip a cloth into the solution to wipe away areas that are likely to be prone to body smells.

5. This could be caused by the food you eat. Avoid eating foods with strong odors like curry, onions and garlic. Limiting your intake oil and fatty food is another important thing to do. The smell and other elements in these food items could penetrate your pores and cause a foul odour.

6. If you are often involved in physically-challenging activities, such as sports and exercises, always change your clothes and

wash them often. Unwashed, sweaty clothes can be a breeding ground of bacteria.

For sensitive skin people, homemade deodorant

Look through many resources to find the perfect deodorant recipe. Be careful when trying different recipes. These deodorants are generally safe. However, your skin may require a different formulation. Some people with sensitive skin found that making their own deodorants led to skin irritations.

Before you get to try out some recipes for sensitive skin, here is a list of common ingredients and possible side effects.

1. Parabens. These chemicals can alter your hormonal balance. It can cause organ and birth defects, as well as toxic effects. They are an artificial preservative that is

often included in many personal care products.

2. Aluminum. This ingredient is found in many store-bought odorants. It has been linked to breast cancer and Alzheimer's diseases in a number of studies. Maximum of

There is no evidence that would support these concerns, but it is better be safe than sorry.

3. Phthalates. They have been linked with birth defects.

4. Propylene glycol. While the petroleum-based chemical is generally safe, it can cause serious damage to your heart, liver, central nervous system, and other organs.

These deodorant recipes are easy to create and safe for people with sensitive skin. Once you're comfortable creating your own homemade deodorant, and you find the right mixtures of ingredients that suit your skin best, you'll enjoy it. It might even prompt you to mix-and-match the ingredients.

Recipe #1: Deodorant Stick for Sensitive Hair

To make this, you will need 3 tablespoons melted beeswax, 2 teaspoons baking soda (note: if your skin is very sensitive, you might reduce the amount to 1 teaspoon), 1/3 Cup coconut oil, 1/3 Cup of Arrowroot powder, 2 Tablespoons of Shea butter, and 15 drops each of your preferred essential oils. Also, keep two empty deodorant containers handy.

You can add any oil you like, but here's a few good suggestions. Oils such as Purification, tea tree, and tea tree are well-known because of their deodorizing abilities. You can add 5 drops each of these oils, and choose from fragrant oils to complete the recipe. For scents, the most preferred ones are lavender and Tangerine. Avoid citrus oils when you are regularly exposed to the sun as they are photosensitive.

First, melt the coconut oil, shea butter, and beeswax in saucepan. Stir everything together until well-combined. Next, remove the pan from the stove. Add the baking soda (arrowroot powder) to the pot. Use a whisk to combine the ingredients. Mix the essential oils in a bowl. You need to mix fast so that the mixture doesn't get too thick. Put the mixture into the containers. Allow the mixture sit for several days. Once your homemade deodorant is set, you are ready to use it.

Be aware that you can now buy beeswax pellets rather than using grated beeswax. It is time-consuming to grind a beeswax strip. It is important to keep the pellets in a handy container so you can grab them easily when making homemade deodorant.

Recipe #2: Natural Deodorant for Sensitive skin

Ingredients: 2 tablespoons baking soda (or 1/3 cup coconut oils and 1/3 cup arrowroot powder. 15 drops essential oils. Prepare a container where the product will be stored, such as a small mason or empty plastic container.

In a bowl, combine the baking soda (and coconut oil) and the arrowroot powder. Mix all of the ingredients together until they are well combined. You can use the back end of the spoon for a similar consistency to a deodorant. Add the essential oils. The other essential oils used in this type recipe include patchouli, sweet orange and cinnamon. There are other options.

Once the mixture has been combined and is of the right consistency, you can transfer it to the container you have prepared using a spoon/spatula. This is it!

Use this homemade deodorant as a rub-on for your underarms. Let them dry for a few minutes before putting on your dress.

Please note that this type of deodorant is likely to melt when it heats up. This is due to the fact that coconut oil is heat-sensitive and melts at high temperatures. The deodorant can still be used, but you can keep it solid by placing the container in the fridge.

FYI

These two recipes work as deodorants, not antiperspirants. Your body will detox naturally through sweating. The deodorant works by stopping bacterial growth. The homemade deodorants won't leave any stains on your shirt as many antiperspirants do. Allow them to dry for a while and then absorb into your armpits.

Basic Homemade Deodorant Recipe

This is the most basic recipe you can use to make your own deodorant. You can make adjustments to the recipe depending on your tolerance and reactions. This is made entirely from natural ingredients and is even edible. It also has antibacterial qualities and moisturises and nourishes the skin.

Recipe #3: The Basic Homemade Odorant Recipe

8 tablespoons Coconut oil (use solidified), 1/4 Cup cornstarch or powder, and 1/4 Cup baking soda.

Mix equal amounts baking soda and any other ingredient you choose between cornstarch or arrowroot. Gradually add in the coconut oil. Use a hand mixer to blend well. Alternatively, you could use a spoon. You want to achieve a consistency that is firm but not too soft, similar in texture to store-bought perfumes. To make it thicker, add more cornstarch (or arrowroot) to make it thicker.

You can either use an empty deodorant container, mason pot or other container with lids to put your homemade concoction. The recipe yields approximately 1 cup of deodorant. This can last for three months if it is used daily by at least two people.

Keep the container cool and dry so it doesn't melt, even in hot weather.

Frequently Asked Questions on Homemade Deodorants

1. Can I use coconut oil as a substitute for other oils

While this is not recommended it is possible. In this example, coconut oil can be substituted with olive oil or sweet, apricot, oil. But the end result will not look the same. Both oil substitutes can be used in place of coconut oil, but they will not work the same way. Palm oil, which is solid at room temp, can be used as another substitute. Coconut oil has more anti-bacterial qualities than other oils, but it is much less.

You can also substitute coconut oil for it with shea butter and cocoa butter, if you are allergic to coconut oils. You can also continue using palm oil. You can also add tea tree essential oil to improve the antibacterial capabilities of the mixture.

2. Is there a certain type of coconut cream I should search for?

A health food store should only sell the highest quality products. Refined coconut oils can be used as a deodorant. This is safer for the skin and more affordable than regular coconut oil. However, this oil cannot be eaten.

3. Which is better, cornstarch and arrowroot powder, to be used in this recipe?

These two ingredients can be used to thicken the mixture. The arrowroot is a substitute for cornstarch in many dishes that use it. It will produce a thicker mixture. The benefit of cornstarch is its easy availability. However, you can buy the arrowroot Powder at your local pharmacy.

4. What are the best essential oils to use in this basic recipe

Essential oils can be used as a way to add aroma. These oils can be used for as long or as you feel you are free from allergic reactions. You can test your skin by doing a small patch. Test a small amount of oil on your skin to determine if you have any adverse reactions. If it does then wash the oil well with water and soap. Tea tree oil emits a unique scent that can be enjoyed by all genders. Many prefer this oil for its antibacterial and pleasant scent.

5. Will the homemade deodorant stain or stain my clothes

It is best to let the deodorant dry completely on your skin before applying your clothes. If ever it does stain your clothes, it will be minimal as compared to the stain that you will get from using the commercially-available types of deodorant and antiperspirant. You can remove the minor stain easily by washing your clothes in warm water and using dishwashing soap.

6. Is it also antiperspirant?

No. While this will not stop you sweating, it will slow down the sweating. Its main purpose is to remove body odor. It is recommended to use this product several times per day for anyone who has been involved in physical exertion.

7. After using it, itchy arms develop. What can be done?

Three factors could explain this phenomenon. One, your body is adapting to it. Two, it also removes impurities which were left behind by your previous antiperspirant. After about a week of continuous use, the condition should disappear. If it doesn't, your skin may react to baking soda. You can reduce baking soda's amount by half and add cornstarch or more arrowroot. The third reason is to not apply the deodorant immediately after shaving. It is recommended that you wait for at least two hours before applying the odorant.

Aloe Vera gel, or juice, can be applied to your armpits prior to applying the deodorant. Aloevera has cooling properties and can make you feel fresh and cool.

The Main Ingredients & Your Choices for Essential Oils

There are many homemade deodorant ideas that you can find at different places. This is one example of how more people are interested and trying out this natural product. This product is also less expensive. It can be difficult to use at first as you have to ensure that your skin is not sensitive or allergic.

Here are the main ingredients needed to make homemade deodorants. There are two types: one that contains all these and the other that has a combination of all three.

Coconut Oil

Coconut oil is rich in antibacterial qualities. Coconut oil can come in many forms including unrefined, virgin and raw coconut oils. The oil can be liquefied at temperatures up to 76 degrees. It can be kept solid in temperatures below 76°C.

Coconut oil offers many benefits to your skin. It has vitamins E, oils, proteins, antiaging elements, and saturated fatty acids that make the skin feel soft. This oil is also effective in treating skin conditions, such as eczema, acne, and psoriasis. Further studies are ongoing to verify the claims about other health benefits such as the ability to replace dying cells by healthy ones and the ability to fade any visible marks or other skin damage.

Almond Oil

The coconut oil and this can be added to the mix to make the product more fluid. It contains good amounts of vitamins A, D, E and F, essential minerals and antioxidants, healthy fats, protein, and healthy fats. This is why coconut oil is so widely used in many skin products.

Baking soda

It works by removing odors. But if you are sensitive to it, bake soda should be used in very small quantities.

Arrowroot Powder

This ingredient is often used in skin care recipes. It makes the mixture more dense and, once it is added to your deodorant it helps to eliminate any toxins. It also moisturizes and clears skin. It can also have a rejuvenating affect on your skin.

Cornstarch

It is soothing to apply on your skin.

Shea Butter

You can use either unrefined, or raw shea Butter. Both are rich in vitamins A & E. It has a soothing effect on the skin.

Beeswax

The raw type of honeywax is used to stabilize the mixture. This can be used in many kinds skin care products. It can moisturize the skin and doesn't clog pores.

Diatomaceous Earth(DE)

It is important to have this handy. It can be used indoors or outdoors to remove insects and fleas. It contains silica, which is beneficial for skin as it helps draw out toxins.

Vitamin E

It has antioxidant and healing qualities. It is a popular ingredient in many beauty care and skin care products.

Natural Oils for Your Skin Type

Many essential oils can also be bought online. You can buy them in either bottles or capsules. Select the oils that suit your skin type when choosing essential oils that you can use in your homemade deodorant recipe.

Normal Skin

This type of skin is neither dry nor oily. You can use all types of oils in this situation. You do not need to pick the type of oil. Oils can be chosen based on how their scents affect your mood. Jasmine (or peppermint) or lavender are good options if you're looking for oils that have an uplifting smell. Rosewood (geranium), rosewood, Cedarwood (soy), orange, tea tree oil and evening primrose are other oils that make you feel good.

Oily Skin

This kind of skin responds best to Ylang–ylang. The oil balances the glands which produce sebum. Melisa can be used in place of ylangylang.

Combination Skin

This is the skin that most people have. Lavender is a top choice for its soothing and healing qualities. It also smells fantastic. Other oils such as rose Geranium Hydrosol, rosewood or ylang–ylang, geranium or neroli hydrosol can also be used.

Dry and Aging skin

Rosehip oil for dry skin is a popular choice. This oil is used in many skin care products. It contains vitamin A as well as essential fatty acids omega 3 to 6. It can help heal your skin. It can treat scarring and acne.

This oil has great hydrating and anti-aging properties. The oil can be used as a deodorant and in liquid baths or body creams. For this skin type, you can use ylang-ylang and geranium oils.

Sensitive skin

It takes some trial and error to identify which oils your skin is sensitive. Rose is the most safest choice, even though it can be more expensive than other oils. This oil can also be used to make moisturizers and facial creams. Other oils that can be used on the skin include angelica, jasmine and rosewood.

Skin with Eczema & Dermatitis

Jasmine essential oil can be a good recommendation for those with skin conditions like these. These oils have soothing and healing effects that are highly effective for treating skin problems like this.

Acne-Prone Skin

Look for oils that can fight bacteria and help with skin conditions. Frankincense is the best option.

Check out these more homemade deodorant recipes

This chapter will cover the three types you can make of deodorants: a spray-on, a spray on and a solid. These deodorants don't contain baking sugar, which can lead to allergic reactions.

Recipe #4: All-Natural Deodorant Stick

For this to happen, you'll need 3 tablespoons Virgin Coconut Oil (wet-milled), three tablespoons Baking Soda, two tablespoons Arrowroot powder or Cornstarch, two tablespoons Shea Butter, and a few drops from your preferred essential oil.

The coconut oil and shea butter should be melted in a double-boiler over a medium flame. Mix together until well-combined. It is important to stir the mixture often to ensure uniform oil distribution. Once it has melted, turn off heat. Mix the baking soda, arrowroot powder and cornstarch in to the mixture. Mix it quickly and thoroughly as the mixture becomes more dense as it cools.

A couple of drops of essential Oil can be added. You should not use too much essential oils. It can lead to a strong scent. Before adding oils to the mixture make sure your skin is sensitive. You can make yourself smell fresh with oils such as eucalyptus or lemon balm, Cedarwood, bergamots, patchouli and frankincense.

As long as the container has a lid, you can place the mixture anywhere. Allow the mixture time to cool and harden before closing the lid. To make a stick of deodorant, either pour the mixture in an empty container or use popsicle moulds. A container with a lid can be used to easily apply the deodorant to your underarms. The deodorant stick can is simpler to use as you need to only rub it in your armpits.

If you're using popsicle molds to store the mixture, freeze them for one hour or until they are set. To prevent deodorant sticks from melting, wrap them in wax paper. The finished products should be stored in a dry, cool place. The deodorant could melt or become too soft in hot weather. They should be stored in the fridge until they have solidified. It is best to not keep these in the refrigerator for too much time as it will cause them to become too hard.

Recipe #5 Spray on Deodorant

This all-natural, natural deodorant recipe does NOT contain baking soda. This recipe calls for only four ounces Magnesium oil and up 15 drops of your choice essential oil.

Magnesium oil may be purchased online or from your local health store. But you can also make the oil yourself. Make your own magnesium oil using half a cup each of magnesium flakes or distilled waters. The magnesium chloride flakes should be placed in a heatproof bowl. Boil water to make distilled water. Once this is done, add the boiling hot water to the bowl with the other ingredient. Let cool, then mix well. Once the mixture has cooled down, add the essential oils you prefer and stir.

Combine the mixture in an airtight container. It doesn't require special storage requirements. You can store it in your toilet so you can use it immediately after you have finished taking a hot shower. Be sure to empty out the contents of the container before it reaches the bottom. If there is a little liquid in the bottle, it may contain more essential oil that the magnesium oil. This way, you might still get stingy armpits from the liquid, especially if it's used right after shaving. Be sure to replenish the contents immediately.

Recipe #6 - Baking Soda No-Nonsense Deo

Here's what you need for this recipe: 30g coconut oils, 10g honey, 15g food grade diatomaceous soil, 20g shea butter.

Mix the coconut oil. Mix all ingredients together slowly and repeatedly, stirring frequently. The beeswax takes the longest time to melt of all the oils. Continue stirring until you have a well-combined mixture that is melted. If you don't own a double stove, you can use a large and heat-proof jar to store all the ingredients. Place the water in saucepan and bring to boil. When the water boils, take out the jar. Wait for everything to melt before you take the jar off the heat.

Let the mixture cool slightly on low heat. Next, add the vitaminE (break the capsule for the oil), arrowroot paste, diatomaceous soil and your chosen essential oils to the mixture. Combine all the ingredients in a bowl.

You can also pour the final product into a small jar. It's ready to go once it has cooled down and solidified. Rub your hands with the deodorant, and then rub it into your armpits. You can also put the mixture in popsicle pans. Let them cool for at least one hour before wrapping each one in wax paper.

Deos are now passé

Egyptians used deodorants differently to us today. They were much more difficult and less effective than we are. To mask unpleasant odors they would take an aromatic bath. Then, they would apply scented oils underneath their arms. If combined with regular bathing and the application strong perfumes, shaving underarm hair results in a reduction of body odor. Because it prevented bacteria growth from the armpit, shaving succeeded. However, this was only discovered by scientists later. Egyptians also used perfumed butter to their heads. The fat releases a pleasant scent as it melts.

Natural deodorants have a wonderful reputation.

Mineral salts were once used to clean the armpit. It was widely used in Asia and is still a popular practice. Because of their long-held reputation as an excellent and safe deodorizer, these body-odor-eliminating mineral salts today form the basis of many current natural deodorants.

Not interested in maintaining a clean home

Personal hygiene and deodorant was not something that was important to Viking-era England. John Wallingford an English Cleric says that the Vikings combed their hair daily, washed on Saturdays, and changed clothes frequently to help them undermine the virtues in married English ladies, and even lure the daughters to be their mistresses. So, we can only imagine how filthy everyone else was. The Viking bath that was held every Saturday is very unhygienic. You might think, "It sounds like certain people from history don't like being cleaned," and you would be right. Napoleon, French Emperor, was said to be writing to Josephine, "J'arrive. "Do Not Launder" means "I'll Be Home Soon." Do not wash!"

Deodorant of Present

Deo in its current commercial form is newer than ever. MUM was the first commercial deodorant. This cream was made with the fingertips and was invented in 1888. MUM's creators developed the roll-on method of application after being inspired to do so by the Ball-Point Pen. EverDry (the first antiperspirant) was introduced in 1903. EverDry was so strong that it ate through fabrics. Antiperspirants of today can leave yellow stains at the armpits, which can cause serious damage to clothing.

Aerosole and Stick Antiperspirants/Deodorants

In the 1950s aerosol antiperspirants (and deodorants containing aluminum zinc and chlorofluorocarbon propellers (CFCs), became available. These aerosol deodorants are hugely popular and account for over 80% in total deodorant sales. Aluminum zirconium was banned by the FDA in 1977. This was due to serious concerns about the health effects that this substance could have on the lungs. The

Environmental Protection Agency discouraged chlorofluorocarbon propellers because of its potential to damage the Ozone layer. However, many people still have questions about the safety of deodorants or antiperspirants.

Stick deodorants or antiperspirants have been popular since the 1970s.

Natural Deos are still available today

Natural deodorants, which are safe and sustainable alternatives to conventional deodorants, have been growing in popularity. Natural deodorants can be made from the same salts used in ancient Asia. The deodorant's salt does not restrict the natural sweating process by constricting pores. Instead, it prevents scent from being formed by limiting the growth bacteria. Crystal Spring's Salt of the Earth products are non-obtrusive and do not leave white streaks on clothing. They are non-toxic to your environment, contain no CFCs and have never been tested on animals.

What is the Difference between Antiperspirant & Deo?

Antiperspirants, deodorants, and others can help reduce body odor. Antiperspirants decrease sweat production. Deodorants are able to raise the skin's pH.

According to the Food and Drug Administration (FDA), deodorants can be considered cosmetic. A product that is designed to cleanse and enhance the skin. Antiperspirants can be described as a drug by the FDA: A substance that is used to treat, prevent, or modify the structure or function the body.

Continue reading for details about the differences in these two types, and which one is more suitable for you.

Deodorants

Deodorants have a dual purpose: to reduce sweat production and odor in the armpits. They are often based on alcohol. They reduce the appeal of microorganisms and acidify your skin when they are applied.

Perfume is often added to deodorants in order to mask odor.

Antiperspirants

The active ingredients in antiperspirants include aluminum-based chemicals that temporarily block the flow of sweat. Blocked sweat pores will reduce the amount perspiration that reaches the skin.

If OTC (over-the-counter) antiperspirants have failed to regulate your sweat, prescription antiperspirants will be offered.

Advantages of Deo and Antiperspirant

You should use deodorants or antiperspirants for moisture and odor control.

Moisture

Sweating acts as a cooling function and allows us heat to be expelled. The sweat gland density is higher in the armpits than elsewhere in the body. Some people want to reduce their sweating since armpit perspiration can sometimes seep under clothing.

Sweating can also cause odor.

Smell

Perspiration does have a stench, but it is not caused by the sweat itself. The smell is due to microorganisms living on your skin. Your armpits are warm and moist for bacteria.

Sweat from your Aporine glands, found in your armpits or groin area, is rich protein that bacteria can readily digest.

Natural Deodorant - Why Choose It?

I first started searching for natural deodorant to get rid of the horrible ingredients in conventional deodorants. But, it has remained a constant favorite since I discovered that it works!

No, I'm serious! Secret Clinical Strength was released right before prom one year ago. Since switching to natural, I've only used it a few times and it doesn't work nearly as well. Although it is not antiperspirant like other deodorants, it seems to retain a lot of moisture.

After just a few months of usage, an unanticipated side effect of natural products began to emerge. I didn't work up a sweat at all. Months later, it's still there.

It's a great idea to play around with the ingredients in your deodorant. Even though you might not care about the ingredients, wouldn't it be nice to know that your deodorant is safe for you and your skin? You can try it out if that's what you decide. Please share your story with me!

Antiperspirants increase the risk of developing breast cancer

Active ingredients of antiperspirants that are made up of aluminum-based chemicals prevent sweat from reaching the skin by inhibiting sweat glands.

There is concern that aluminum compounds may alter estrogen receptors in breasts if they are absorbed through their skin.

But, the American Cancer Society asserts that there's no clear link between antiperspirants (and cancer) and aluminum.

Breast cancer tissue doesn't appear to have higher levels of aluminum than normal tissue.

A study on antiperspirants which contain aluminum chlorohydrate revealed that only a trace amount was absorbed (0.0012%).

Additional studies suggesting no link between breast and underarm product use include:

A 2002 study of 793 women without breast cancer history and 813 with breast cancer showed that women who used antiperspirants and deodorants in the armpits were at no higher risk for breast cancer.

A 2006, smaller-scale investigation corroborated 2002's findings.

A systematic review published 2016

A reliable source

PubMed Central is an abbreviation of PubMed Central

The National Institutes of Health boasts a highly regarded database.

You can go to the source

Although it was not possible to link breast cancer risk with antiperspirant abuse, the study suggested that further research is needed.

Although sweating can occur, your sense of smell does not.

Burpees performed on crowded trains, delivering presentations, and riding on trains can all be dangerous for your underarms. The majority of antiperspirants and traditional deodorants work by reducing body odor and moisture.

But the chemicals used can make your pits stink and could even be harmful. They can even alter the pH level in your pits to create bacteria friendly sweat saunas.

We offer information about natural deodorants.

What causes pet stink? And how does deodorant work?

BO's science is disturbing. Our underarms, much like a petri-dish from middle school, provide a warm habitat for bacteria. These guys eat our moisture as we perspire. Their munching creates the smell of sweat.

While deodorants and antiperspirants serve separate purposes, many pit sticks on the market are deodorant-antiperspirant combinations. Traditional deodorants kill microorganisms via antimicrobial substances or ethanol. Antiperspirants, by contrast, use aluminum based salts that clog sweat glands to stop armpit bugs feeding and stinking up.

This might sound tempting to you. Not so quickly. A 2016 study showed that traditional cosmetics have a negative impact on the ecosystem of your skin. You might be contributing to your body's odor and weakening your immune systems. Corynebacterium were found in the bottoms of study participants, even those who had not used pit product. This bacterium can not only cause BO but can also help humans fight infection.

Staphylococcus, Propionibacterium, Corynebacterium and Micrococcus all exist in the armpit. It is normal to have some microorganisms in your skin.

Some bacteria, including those found in the gut, can be beneficial. However, antiperspirants can encourage the growth and introduction of new germs. These germs could be more stinky than they were before.

You can make a deo that goes with your chemistry

Natural products can be a great alternative to the traditional stick if you want to increase your pit bacteria. These deodorants do not contain synthetic ingredients. They often include the following three components:

Other components that possess antibacterial and/or disinfecting characteristics such as coconut oil, tea tree oil, or olive oil are also available.

Essential oils such as lavender, sandalwood or bergamot will give off a pleasing scent.

For moisture resistance, you can use naturally absorbent substances like cornstarch, baking soda, and arrowroot.

Natural deodorants will not clog your sweat glands like other antiperspirants. Additionally, they won't contain aluminum as an ingredient, which is a frequent cause of concern.

Natural deodorants mask odor and not perspiration. This is a good thing.

It is not possible to predict how natural deodorants will perform when you change from conventional deodorants. It could take several hours or even weeks for your ecosystem to recover from natural deodorants. To speed up the process, you could try an armpit cleansing. However, natural deodorants are not designed to stop sweating. They'll try to reduce odor when temperatures rise.

We don't want any loss of our unique smell signature. It isn't a bad thing that body odor is referred to as. Although our eyes are where physical attraction is strongest, our noses have a significant impact on who we choose and when.

Your natural, exposed scent is perfectly acceptable in every day situations, even though it might be difficult to go on dates without taking a hot yoga class. This is one of your most desirable characteristics.

Let nature have its way

Natural deodorant may be purchased in any health food store that sells natural skin-care items, as well online. The following products are among the most sought-after:

Schmidt's Organic Deodorant

Green Tidings natural deodorant unscented

Pit Paste (Primal)

The process of finding the best natural deodorant might not be easy. This could be like trying to find your favorite pair. Because everyone smells differently, it is also because we smell different.

According to a 2013 study each one of us has a unique genetic collection that leads to different ways we perceive odors. It may be unpleasant for you to see how your natural scent interacts with a stick with patchouli. However, it might be a delight for your sister to see how it interacts and interacts with her chemistry. Explore different natural deodorants, until you find one you love.

You can customize your deodorant.

You can also make your own online selections if they don't suit you. This simple recipe is your guide:

Ingredients:

34 cups of coconut oil

Use a quarter of a cup of baking powder

1 tbsp arrowroot starch

Add 6-10 drops to essential oils, if desired.

Instructions:

Combine the baking soda in with the arrowroot.

Blend in the coconut oils until smooth. If desired, add essential oils.

You can fill a half-full glass container with the mixture.

To make it liquid, heat a small amount between your fingertips. Use this on your pits.

Make your own natural perfume by mixing powders, oils and bases. While base options like shea and coconut oils, as well as bases such cocoa butter and shea oil, work well. You don't always need to use one, if all you want is a powdered mix. Add equal amounts of baking powder and arrowroot to the mix, then add your oil choice and shake it up. Use the mixture in a small spice jar.

Your sense of smell is also affected by your diet.

These BO hacks may be helpful if you're using natural deodorant and still have problems with body odor. Consider what you eat. A 2006 study of 17 men showed that eating red meat may affect our ability to smell. You might be surprised at the impact certain foods have on your breath. These meals may make your whole body smell stronger, especially if you're sweating.

Talk to your doctor about any concerns you have regarding your stench. Odoriferousness may be exacerbated by certain illnesses and medical conditions.

Remember that sweating and body odors are natural. Don't let your arms prevent you from lifting your hands up in the air and having some fun.

How to make your day smell good

The essence of smelling great boils down into what you consider a pleasant aroma.

One person's idea of being nice is to bring a delicate French perfume with them everywhere they go. It could be that someone doesn't get sweaty after a long work day.

We'll show your how to scent like perfume, or just your natural self, and how to make it last throughout the day.

Keep your perfume and cologne on the scene for as long as possible.

A little perfume goes far. If you use the fragrance correctly, it can help you get the most enjoyment.

Use it on the pulse points. This allows your body chemistry to organically react with the scent. Your body will heat up and ignite the scent. Be careful not to rub the scent on your skin.

A roll-on version is best. A rollerball can be used to apply fragrance exactly where you want without having it sprayed too heavily. It's also cheaper than buying a bottle your favorite perfume or fragrance.

Apply to a brush. Spray your hairbrush using your favorite fragrance to give it a long-lasting scent.

You should spray the following pulse locations:

The back of your throat

Know all the places where your elbows are located

Your biceps

Your back should be behind you.

Amazon and Sephora offer roll-on perfumes. You can also purchase an online funnel to help you pour your favorite scent into a rollerball jar.

You can moisturize your skin by using creams and perfumed lotions.

If your favorite perfume, cream or oil lasts a long time, apply it right after you've dried off the water.

If scented lotions are put on a moist foundation, they last longer.

Do you desire to add a little bit of fragrance? Make sure to use lotions, creams, and other products from the same manufacturer that make your favorite scents. These items can be layered by shave creams, shower gel, or perfumes that are complementary.

Shower and then get to the right spots

The scent of your body's perfume has a lot do with hygiene. However, genetics as well as what you eat can have an influence on the way your body smells.

Genetics are out of your control. There are many things you can't control, including the odor-producing items like garlic, broccoli, and fish. But they are delicious and healthy. Cleanliness, however, can be managed.

Shower frequency depends on the skin type, activity levels, and personal preference. Shower once per day. Do not wash your skin fast. Instead, focus on the areas where you have the most sweat glands.

armpits \sgroin \sbutt

Use an antiperspirant (deodorant)

You can also do:

Use deodorant or antiperspirant, and have a portable version for those sweaty days.

For a quick and easy way to stay hydrated, keep a few individually wrapped wipes handy. Online ordering is possible for travel wipes.

Apply talc-free, powdered talc to areas where your skin rubs together.

Avoid polyester. Polyester has been shown to trap sweat and bacteria in studies, which can cause unpleasant stench.

How to keep hair fresh and healthy throughout the day

The instructions on the shampoo bottle for lathering, rinse, then repeat are not to be ignored. Every time you turn your heads, your hair will smell amazing after you have cleaned it.

The Academy of Dermatology suggests that shampoo be concentrated on the scalp before being applied to the rest of your hair.

A decent shampoo removes oil and debris from the scalp. It can leave your hair feeling less shampoo-fresh.

How to keep your breath fresh and clean throughout the day

Bad oral hygiene is the most common cause of bad breath. But, even though you take great care of your teeth, an occasional foul odor could still sneak in.

Here are some tips and tricks to keep you breath fresh throughout your day.

To maintain your health, brush your mouth twice a day, each time for two seconds.

You should floss once daily to remove food particles from between your teeth.

After eating meals that contain strong scents such as garlic, onions and tuna you need to brush your teeth.

Hydration is key to preventing dry mouth which can lead a foul odor.

You can get rid naturally of foul breath by chewing fresh mint leaves

You can always keep gum or sugar-free mints handy in an emergency.

Avoid fragranced products

Take a hot shower and say goodbye to the day.

The clean, delicate scent of soap or bodywash is appealing. It's also possible to use soaps without fragrance or unscented body wash.

After applying the lotion, allow yourself to soak in the water for a couple of minutes. After washing your hands, rinse all sweaty areas like the armpits.

How to keep clothes fresh throughout the day

Washing clothes frequently is the easiest way to keep them smelling fresh. There are a variety of fragrance boosters that may be added to the wash to enhance the fresh-from-the-laundry smell.

Try these alternatives:

Use Febreze or linen spray as a fabric odorant to freshen your clothes.

Use 10 to 20 drops oil in your wash.

Add a few drops of borax to the water and mix it with some baking soda.

Make sachets or hang dry lavender in your wardrobe.

Consider filling your drawers in cotton balls or tissue papers scented with your favorite scent.

Chapter 19: Deodorant: What is it?

Sweating is an effective way for the body to eliminate toxins. Most people, regardless of their genes, have worn deodorant at some point in their lives. Bet you've tried everything, from roll-on liquids to body sprays, deo-sticks, and even body sprays. However, all of them failed after a hard workout or long day on the job. Body odor is something many people are uncomfortable discussing, but we all have been there.

In addition, antiperspirants and other deodorants have been shown to cause cancers and Alzheimer's disease. As you can see, online communities are increasingly interested in developing an all natural, non-toxic deodorant.

Due to bacteria in our armpits, we often have body odor. Commercial antiperspirants block sweat from exiting the body. The problem with conventional deodorants is that they don't reduce sweating. They also cause skin to become acidic which makes it more vulnerable for odor-generating bacteria.

Commercial Deodorant: There Are Some Risks

All deodorants, no matter what form, contain aluminum derivatives. Even those deodorants that claim to have "all natural" ingredients have been linked to the development and spread of other chronic diseases, such as breast cancer, and others. Parabens make up the majority of deodorants, face creams, and lotions. They help prolong product shelf life. Petroleum is where it comes from. Parabens can lead to estrogen-related problems, malfunctioning endocrine system, and even cancer.

Parabens can also cause allergic reaction. It is important that you note that handmade deodorants will not contain harsh chemicals like commercial deodorants.

Additional ingredients like triclosan could make the underarm skin too acidic and/or salty. They also contain wax (or other aluminum-based chemical) which is an active component that provides antiperspirants' sweat-blocking capabilities.

Why go natural?

Many people love the branded cosmetics and beauty products. However, others want to live healthier lives and use all-natural and organic products. Others wanted to avoid getting certain health diseases by using products that have many chemicals. While your natural deodorant may not work, this doesn't mean you need to stop using it. Just do more research and play with other ingredients.

We urge you create your own deodorant.

What to Use in Your Deo

Here are some common and useful ingredients to make natural antiperspirants.

Coconut Oil and Almond Oil. Coconut Oil is known for its antibacterial properties. This oil is essential for your armpits. A combination of coconut oil and almond oils helps to liquefy or give the deodorant its semisolid state.

Beeswax, we've all heard of honey being a fantastic ingredient in beauty product formulations. It seems that beeswax makes it into the top ten list of ingredients. It doesn't clog pores and keeps oils in your skin locked in, so it won't clog them.

Beeswax also has the ability to stick to skin, making it waterproof. This will thicken your product, and it will also give it a sweet smell. It is important to be cautious with beeswax, particularly if you got it from the store. Beeswax with a yellow or white color is already processed and may contain chemical compounds. Avoid buying beeswax from stores and look for other natural sources.

Nature provides us with another wonderful gift, Shea Butter or Cocoa Butter. Raw Shea butter, which is unrefined and unprocessed, is rich in vitamins E and A. It is also known to soothe the skin. It has an extremely creamy texture with a pleasant sweet scent.

The cocoa butter is oilier, less dense and has the moisturizing effects Shea butter. Cocoa beans that are used to make cocoa butter also contain healing properties. Cocoa beans must be unrefined and organic to reap their nutritional benefits.

Arrowroot Powder can also be used in your deodorant recipe. It can also be used to make food and skincare recipes.

Arrowroot powder may increase the product's thickness, while drawing out toxins.

You should cleanse your body first before using any type deodorant, antiperspirants, or other products. Before you use deodorants, be sure to wash your arms. Or else, you'll only be making the problem worse. Sweating, while natural and healthy, is beneficial to our overall health.

Chapter 20: Detox the Armpits Firstly

Make sure you cleanse your arms before we begin with our natural deodorants recipes. This will make natural deodorants more effective. It can speed up the adjusting of your skin. At the same time it helps in pulling out any harsh chemicals in your armpit skin from years of using conventional deodorants.

For the ingredients:

1 tbsp. Bentonite pottery

1 tsp. 1 teaspoon.

2 tbsps. 2 tbsps.

Mix all ingredients into a glass. To avoid chemical reactions, don't use a metallic container. Mix the ingredients by using a wooden spoon (or any non-metal tool).

Allow the mixture to settle for between 10-20minutes. It is important to immediately relieve any pain you feel. Although it can cause some redness due to increased blood flow, it will quickly disappear. Then rinse with warm water.

If you are used to using chemical-laden deodorants or antiperspirants, it is common for you to experience sensitive detox. Some people feel rashes and pain in the arms after detoxification. In the interim, you may want to spray colloidal silver. This will keep you from getting stale and help heal your rashes quicker.

Other than using hand-made deodorant and detoxifying your armpits with it, it's important to eat a balanced healthy diet. This will help eliminate bad odor. Make sure you drink plenty water.

Why Some People Feel Sick

Sorry for the pun, but many people are still afflicted by that foul-smelling smell, even though they regularly wash and bathe. No matter what deodorant we use, there will be times when we still smell. Here are some common reasons why people sometimes stink even though they are tidy and clean.

Food intolerance - According to some health professionals, food intolerance (inability to properly assimilate or digest foods) can make someone smell. Some people believe that lactose can also cause unpleasant odors, particularly for people who cannot tolerate dairy products. There may be food intolerances you don't know about.

Try to reduce your wheat and dairy intakes for a couple of week. Examine whether you notice any changes in the way your smells.

Hormonal disturbance - Body odor may be caused by hormonal imbalances, especially for women. To rule out such an imbalance, you should have your hormones checked first.

Try it without deodorant. This is a good option if you are at home and have nothing to do that will require you to sweat. The body can't naturally eliminate toxins from the skin because most commercial deodorants hinder its ability to sweat. If you notice that you are sweating but not stinking, then you might have an allergic reaction with the ingredients in your deodorant.

Sensitive reactions can occur when homemade deodorants include baking soda, cornstarch or other food ingredients. These ingredients can make people smell musty. To minimize the smell, you can replace baking soda with powdered arrowroot.

Too much sugar can be detrimental to our health. Reduce your intake of all types of sugar to notice the difference.

Chapter 21: Deodorant For Sensitive skin

Some handmade deodorants can irritate skin with sensitive armpits. Due to the harsh chemicals, conventional deodorants can produce the same results.

Natural deodorant is still the best option. It has food ingredients which are safer and it's also cheaper to make. It is important to maintain a balanced pH. Too much acid may cause skin irritations in the armpits. Women's pH levels are generally slightly lower than men's, but they remain within the same range (from 5.5-7.2). There are deos that contain too many alkaline ingredients, so there is a special deo to suit those with sensitive skin.

Detox Reactions Possible

Sometimes, pH is not a problem. The liver is the main detox pathway of our body. The liver works alongside the kidneys, colon, lymph system and skin to detoxify or get rid of toxins. So, using a conventional deodorant, which contains aluminum, parabens, triclosan, and aluminum, in your armpits will cause the skin to not do its job. Make sure to clean out your armpit before you can use homemade deodorant.

Allergic Reaction

Food allergies and food sensitivities can make it more difficult to be allergic to handmade deos. Below is the recipe for a soothing and gentle deodorant.

This gentle baking soda formula is great for sensitive people. Diatomaceous Earth - Have you ever heard of it? It is a powdered form of fossilized phytoplankton. This product is very microbial, high in silica. Its pH will vary depending on the source. However, it is usually lower than that of baking soda.

Diatomaceous Earth also makes a great ingredient for household products such as toothpaste and exfoliating scrubs. This ingredient can also be used in handmade deodorants to pamper your armpits, as well as draw out harmful toxins.

For the ingredients:

3/cup cornstarch and/or Arrowroot powder

1/4 cup diatomaceous (food grade)

5-8 tbsp coconut butter (melted).

Combine the cornstarch/arrowroot powder and diatomaceous clay in a small container. Use a whisk to mix the coconut oil. Depending on the consistency that you are looking for, you may add more coconut oils. Use a clean container with a tight cap or lid to place the mixture.

The same as with handmade deodorants, you may also directly apply the mixture to your armpits if necessary.

Recipe #2 with Shea Butter und Bentonite Ceramic

Here is another recipe that makes a non-toxic, natural deodorant.

5 tbsp. Arrowroot powder

2-3 tablespoons Shea butter

2 Tbsp melted coconut butter

2-3 tbsp. Bentonite and Clay

Choose an essential oil

Bentonite Clay can be used to heal and is considered to be the most effective. Experts state that it has a strong, negative charge which bonds with toxic substances. The clay is also capable of absorbing toxic chemicals and heavy metals as well as its own minerals. Bentonite aids in oxygen flow to cells.

Bentonite clay has a non-staining and pleasant odor, which makes it a good option for natural deodorant. It absorbs sweat and moisture quickly to stop odors.

Combine the coconut oil & Shea butter using a stand mixer. After combining the ingredients, lower your mixer and slowly incorporate the essential oils. In a separate bowl combine all the dry ingredients. Add 1/3 of your mixture of dried ingredients to the first mixture.

Slowly add the remaining ingredients. Mix thoroughly. The finished product should be dough-like. This is normal. You can transfer the mixture to another container and seal it. Keep it out of direct heat. Use the mixture as needed. You can also take some in smaller containers.

You should note that while the paste mixture can thicken upon transferring it to room temperatures, it will'melt quickly' when applied to your armpit. It will then absorb easily into your skin.

Coconut Oil and Baking Soda Deo

Coconut oil is a popular ingredient in homemade deodorants.

For the ingredients:

1/3 cup baking powder

1/2 cup of Arrowroot Powder (available from supermarkets or health food stalls).

5 tablespoons Organic Coconut Oil

Grapefruit or lavendar essential oil

Simply mix all ingredients in a medium container until you have the consistency you desire. If you prefer, you may add the essential oils. To use the mixture, you can use either a small jar of a container with a cover or a container. You can use your hands, or a sharp knife or clean stick to apply the deodorant. As long it is safe for you and your family, you can use any amount. To avoid smudges from your clothing, wait at most 2 minutes before you start putting it on.

It is important to store your handmade deodorant in a cool location as coconut oil can easily melt making it oily. You can add more baking powder to the mixture. However, if sensitive skin is present, decrease the baking soda.

If your deodorant takes longer for it to harden try putting it in the fridge for about two hours.

Apart from deodorant, it can be used as a homemade toothpaste, facial product, or hair treatment. By researching, you can improve this formula. This will help you gain a better understanding about organic deodorants.

Coconut Oil & Shea Butter Deo

Here's a list of ingredients

3 tbsp coconut butter (raw or virgin)

2-3 tbsp Shea butter

3 tbsp baking salt or 2 teaspoons cornstarch

Drops containing essential oils (such lavender, Chamomile or orange)

Put half a glass water in a small pan and allow it to boil. Heat the coconut oil, Shea butter and coconut butter in a small saucepan until they have melted. After the mixture has melted turn off the heat. Add the cornstarch, baking soda or both. Blend the mixture until smooth. Mix in a few drops essential oil. Let it cool.

Your homemade deodorant can be kept in the fridge during summer so that it doesn't become too oily. You can also use used deodorant bottles to make it easy to apply the mixture.

Chapter 22: Homemade Fragrant Deodorants

Many of us want deodorants or antiperspirants that have a pleasant or refreshing smell. Below are some quick deo recipes that will not only keep your arms fresh, but also leave them sweetly scented!

Cocoa Butter & coconut Oil Deodorant

This recipe can be used on all skin types. Coconut oil and cocoa Butter are good at masking body odors. Just use 1 tbsp. beeswax (organic), 1/2 tsp. cocoa butter (organic), and 1 Tbsp. virgin coconut oils. Pure castor oil and essential oils of rosemary or thyme can be used as well.

The organic cocoa butter, beeswax and honey should be melted in a double boiler. Once it has melted in a double boiler, leave the mixture to cool. Once the mixture is cooled, add coconut oil, castor and other essential oils. Transfer the mixture into a empty deodorant stick.

Mango Butter and Beeswax

You can also make a refreshing deodorant with mango butter, beeswax or pure coconut oil. This recipe yields about 1/2 cup of each mango butter, honey, and beeswax. You will also need 1/2 cup arrowroot powder, 2 tbsp baking flour, ylangylang essential oil, and 2-3 tbsp vitamin E oil.

Mix the coconut oil, mango butter and beeswax together in a double-boiler. Let it cool down slightly once the ingredients are melted. Mix in the arrowroot powder, baking powder, and salt. Then, add the vitamin e oil and ylang-ylang essential oil according to your preference. Mix the ingredients in a container.

Glycerin and grape seed oil

This recipe is for you if essential oils are something you enjoy in your natural products. 1/2 teaspoon of grapeseed oil, 1 teaspoon of baking powder and the essential oils of lavender, peppermint, tea tress, and eucalyptus will be needed.

Simply combine the grapes oil, vegetable glycerin, Shea Butter and Shea butter into a ceramic/glass container. Microwave the mixture for around 10 minutes, or until all ingredients melt. Once the mixture reaches the desired consistency you want, remove it from the microwave and let it cool. The essential oils and baking soda can be added to the mixture.

Citrusy Deodorant

Get a citrusy, fresh scent. This all-natural, natural deo recipe will make you feel fresh and citrusy. 2 tbsp Carnauba wax, 2 Tbsp Bentonite Clay, 5 Tbsp Avocado or Mango Butter, and 5 Tbsp lemongrass essential oils.

Place the avocado or mango butter along with the carnauba honey in a saucepan. Heat on low heat. Stir together the ingredients until they have melted into a paste. Add the bentonite Clay and mix in the rest of your essential oils.

Vitamin E Deo

This one is also amazing, but a little grainy. This recipe requires 3 tbsps each of baking powder and Shea butter. Also, you'll need 2 tbsps Cornstarch, 2 cups of Cocoa butter, 2 cups of cornstarch, two tablespoons of shea butter, and 2 tablespoons each of Vitamin E oil.

All the ingredients are to be melted except for essential oils. Stir until well combined. Add the oils, such as orange or lavender to the mixture and stir again. Mix the ingredients in a bowl and store in a container.

These are some common questions regarding deodorant

What's the solution to itchy underarms when you use homemade deo?

You may feel itchy, irritable or both. This is especially true if you're first using homemade deodorant. The key is to check if your skin has any sensitivities or allergies to ingredients like oils and baking soda. It is best to remove or reduce this ingredient before making your deodorant. Consult your dermatologist to determine if the product suits your needs.

What other oils can I use for my recipe

There are many oils you could substitute for, such as sweet almond oil or sweet apricot butter. But coconut oil is the best oil to use because it has antibacterial properties other oils don't. Coconut oil can also be used in place of other oils, which can make them messy and more difficult to apply. It is therefore a great ingredient for deodorants.

Do I get a stain?

Homemade deodorants tend to be less likely cause staining than standard antiperspirant. For stains less severe than those that are obvious, soak the clothes in hot soapy water with mild detergent.

What is the best type coconut oil to use for cooking?

Choose coconut oil from natural food stores whenever possible to get the best quality. While refined coconut oils can be used, they can be less effective than those made from organic coconut oil.

Can this handmade deodorant cause me to sweat?

Yes. This is exactly what we want. Remember that sweating is your body's natural way to remove toxins.

Therefore, blocking your body's ability of cleaning itself will cause it to stop sweating. It will eventually alter the pH balance and make you more susceptible to infections. You'll still sweat, but it won't make you stink. The majority of homemade deodorants have a very effective effect on masking body odor.

Chapter 23: Soothing Deodorants

Coconut oil is a very popular ingredient in natural deodorants. We will use coconut oil in the next recipe for soothing deo.

Calendula-chamomile Deo

For the ingredients:

Coconut oil, 2-3 tbsp

2 tbsp Calendula rose petals (dried).

3 tbsp. Chamomile (dried).

3 tbsps sunflower essential oil

First, combine the Calendula petals dry and dried Chamomile flower in a jar. Make sure you sterilize it first. For this, you can sterilize it with boiling water. Leave it to cool for 10 minutes. Before you add the ingredients, dry completely the jar. Next, add in the coconut oil. To make it liquefied, you can heat the coconut oil on a low heat. For coconut oil to melt, place it under the sun for at least 15 minutes. Cover the jar with a lid and keep it in a cool place for at least two weeks.

Keep the lid on the jar shaken. After weeks of wait, you will notice that the mixture has turned yellow. Make sure to warm the infused oil. You can either place the jar under the sunlight or put it in a small pot of warm water. The sunflower oil helps to keep the coconut oil hydrated.

Filter the infused olive oil using cheesecloth, coffee filter or paper towel to remove flowers and other floating items. You can make your own mixture.

Some Things to Keep In Mind

Make sure you use a sterilized container for any handmade deodorants.

For those with sensitive skin, Arrowroot powder is a better choice than cornstarch.

If you have allergies, skip chamomile. Calendula, lavender, or ragweed can be used instead.

You should not mix baking powder with baking soda in any of our recipes. You should apply your deodorant stick gently to avoid staining.

Tea Tree Oil Deodorant

Tea tree oil, which has antifungal & antibacterial qualities, is a great ingredient to make homemade deodorant.

These ingredients are available:

Tea tree oil

1/2 cup Baking soda and 1/4 cup Arrowroot powder

5 tbsp Organic Coconut oil

If you don't have arrowroot, you can use cornstarch to replace it. Even though the tea tree oil smells a lot like medicine, it's essential in this recipe. The fragrance will eventually wear off.

Mix the ingredients until it reaches the right consistency. Place the mixture in a small mason or empty deodorant bathtub.

Unscented Homemade Deo Spray

For the ingredients:

2 tbsp aluminum

1 tbsp baking soda

Rubbing alcohol

Mix all the ingredients until they are well combined. Use a spray can to transfer the mixture. Before using, shake the bottle.

Zinc Oxide Perfume

For the ingredients:

1 tbsp powder zinc oxide

1 cup of witchhazel

Aloe Vera juice

Essential oils of choice

In a bowl, combine all the ingredients. Essential oils of rose or lavender may be chosen, as these essential oils can kill bacteria. Mix all ingredients together in a spray bottle. This deodorant works because it contains witch hazel which kills bacteria and inhibits sweat production. The zinc oxide dust helps to neutralize body smells while also adding substance to this formula.

The zinc oxide helps neutralize the odor. It is slightly sticky and will make homemade deodorant appear milky. The powder does not cause skin irritation and has antiseptic qualities. It is important that you shake the solution before using it. Zinc oxide powder is not water-soluble.

Give your body time to adjust to homemade deodorant. You still have many other homemade recipes to try.

Chapter 24: Baking soda - free

Baking soda, while being a very useful ingredient for human health, can cause skin irritations and itching. You don't have to use bake soda in your deodorant.

For the ingredients:

1/2 cup cornstarch/arrowroot paste

Essential oils for tea tree or lavender

1/2 cup organic coconut butter

Drops containing essential oils from lemon, peppermints and orange

The antifungal properties that tea tree oils and lavender oils have are well known. While arrowroot, cornstarch and cornstarch flours work as antiperspirants, the lavender and tea tree oils are also known to be antifungal. Coconut oil can be substituted with other butters if it isn't desired.

Add all the ingredients to a jar. Use your homemade deodorant free from baking soda as often you like. You should keep your homemade deodorant warm so that it doesn't harden.

Bake Soda No-Need Recipe #2

Let's assume you travel often or are currently living in a warm climate. Then you might not like how your deodorant stain clothes or melt in your arms. This second option might be the best.

The ingredients:

2 parts hazel

Aloe vera, 1 part

Essential oils of your choosing

You can combine all ingredients in a spray-bottle. Tea tree oil or rosemary can be used to mask any body odors. Make sure to shake the bottle before you use it. You can also add apple cider vinegar and distilled waters to this recipe. Aloe Vera is a natural cooling agent that will give your finished product its mild cooling effects. It's also known to have remarkable healing and moisturizing properties that will be good for your skin.

Magnesium Oil Deodorant

A magnesium oil spray is an alternative to oil-based deodorants. Although it smells oily, magnesium oils does not contain any oil. Magnesium oils are effective in eliminating underarm odor.

It helps increase your magnesium intake.

If magnesium oil is new to you, some may feel tingling. This is normal and will go away eventually.

These ingredients are available:

Magnesium oils (4 ounces).

Essential oils

Use magnesium oil mixed with your favorite essential oils in a spray bottle. It is better to use a glass bottle, as it will prevent any allergic reaction. You can apply a few drops to your armpit first. If you use the formula after shaving or if it is relatively low in magnesium, expect a stinging sensation.

Baking soda can act in the same way as other food ingredients to cause irritation. This could be your body's way to detoxify your body and eliminate any impurities left over from previous antiperspirants. You can wait a few more weeks to see whether your allergy has disappeared. If it hasn't, you can reduce the baking soda or add other ingredients, such as arrowroot. This is much more natural.

Your deodorant can also be improved by using Shea butter, cocoa butter, or Shea butter. Aloe verde helps reduce irritations and keeps your armpits clean.

Deodorant containing Vodka

Vodka has been gaining popularity in home-made products. Here is another recipe to make it. You'll need 1/8c of Vodka (80proof), 1/4c of distilled or bottled water, and any essential oils.

Mix the vodka with the distilledwater in a jar and then add essential oils. You could use essential oils of rosemary, cypress, or lavender. Gently shake it and then transfer it to the spray bottle. Place this container in a dark and cool place.

Other scent options include sandalwood or anise seeds, geraniums, coriander, coriander, and sage. The deodorant should be used after shaving to create a tingling sensation that will eventually fade.

Witch Hazel Deodorant

This recipe produces an antibacterial scent with essential oils such thyme, clary-sage, and bergamot. A refreshing spray that smells great for both men (and women)

For the ingredients:

1 tsp Vodka

Bergamot essential oils (10 drops)

Clary sage

Rosewood, thyme and rosemary oils

Mandarin and lemon oil

40ml or 4 Tbsp Witch Hazel

25 ml, or 2 tbsp, of linden flowers water

25ml (2 tbsp) orange flower water

Put all of the essential oils in a glass flask. After adding the vodka, shake the bottle vigorously for a few seconds until all oils have been dissolved. Then add the witchhazel to the bottle. To ensure that essential oils are well-mixed, shake the bottle gently before spraying it to your armpit.

But, sage isn't for those with epilepsy or pregnant ladies. Inducing labour is what sage is used for. It can be removed and replaced by other healthier options like chamomile. To avoid irritations, make sure you only use the essential oil mentioned above.

Keep Yourself Fresh

All of these homemade recipes will not prevent you from getting sweaty. Because sweating is essential, that is not what we are trying to achieve. These deodorants work to keep you fresh smelling, no matter what you do.

Underarm shields can be used to protect your clothes from sweating if you are very active. This is a much better alternative to conventional antiperspirants. Perspiration is a natural part of the human body so it should never be hindered. We sweat to help us stay healthy and eliminate toxins.

www.ingramcontent.com/pod-product-compliance
Lightning Source LLC
Chambersburg PA
CBHW060329030426
42336CB00011B/1260